# Sponsors

The 1st Symposium on *Functional Autoantibodies Targeting G-Protein-Coupled Receptors* is kindly supported by

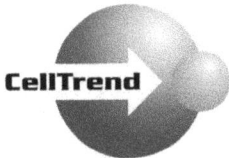

**CellTrend**

Sponsoring: 3000 €

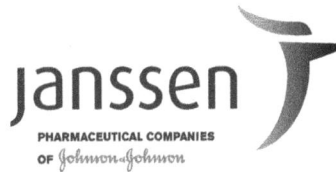

**Janssen**
PHARMACEUTICAL COMPANIES
OF *Johnson&Johnson*

Sponsoring: 2000 €

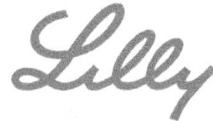

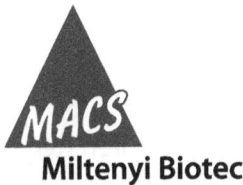

**Bristol-Myers Squibb**

Sponsoring: 2000 €

*Lilly*

Sponsoring: 2000 €

**MACS**
**Miltenyi Biotec**

Sponsoring: 1000 €

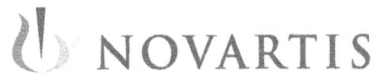

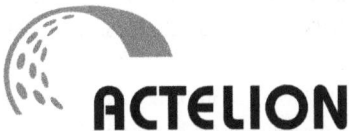

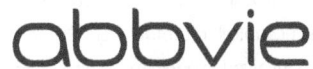

**NOVARTIS**

Sponsoring: 1000 €

**ACTELION**

Sponsoring: 1000 €

**abbvie**

Sponsoring: 700 €

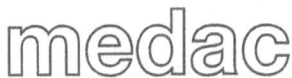

**medac**

Sponsoring: 500 €

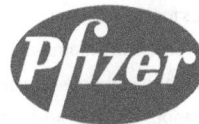

**Pfizer**

Sponsoring: 500 €

**Prof. Dr. Gabriela Riemekasten**
Department of Rheumatology
University of Lübeck
gabriela.riemekasten@uksh.de

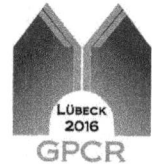

LÜBECK
2016
GPCR

## 1st Symposium on
## Functional Autoantibodies Targeting G-Protein-Coupled Receptors

Greeting from the symposium chair

Dear Sir or Madam, Dear colleagues

It is a great pleasure to announce the first symposium on functional autoantibodies targeting G-protein-coupled receptors (GPCRs) in Lübeck. GPCRs are involved in a variety of physiological and pathophysiological processes. So far, much effort has been made on anti-GPCR drug discovery with a focus on the development of small molecules and monoclonal antibodies for the treatment of cancer, infection, metabolic disorders or inflammatory diseases. Recently, functional autoantibodies against GPCRs were identified in various diseases associated with pathogenesis, uncovering a potential new field of therapeutic intervention. Thus, the aim of this symposium is to combine the current knowledge about the role of GPCRs in different pathologies, their mode of action and state-of-the-art research techniques to identify common fundamental pathways that can be transferred to other disease entities with similar manifestations.

I cordially invite you to participate in this inspiring symposium with outstanding speakers from the field of GPCR research and constructive discussions as well as poster sessions. I look forward to welcome you to the beautiful Hanseatic City of Lübeck and encourage you and your colleagues to contribute to this exciting meeting.

Prof. Dr. Gabriela Riemekasten
- Director, Department of Rheumatology -

**Gabriela Riemekasten**
**and Anja Kerstein (Editors)**

1st Symposium on

**Functional Autoantibodies**
**Targeting G-Protein-Coupled**
**Receptors**

Book of Abstracts

Department of Rheumatology
University of Lübeck

Infinite Science
Publishing

© 2016 Infinite Science Publishing
        University Press and
        Academic Printig

Imprint of Infinite Science GmbH,
MFC 1 | BioMedTec Wissenschaftscampus
Maria-Goeppert-Straße 1
23562 Lübeck

Cover Design: Infinite Science Publishing
Copy Editing: Department of Rheumatology, University of Lübeck and Infinite Science Publishing
Receptor illustration was generated by Anja Kerstein using PDB, OPM database and Jmol

Publisher: Infinite Science GmbH, Lübeck, www.infinite-science.de
Print: Norderstedt, Germany

ISBN Paperback: 978-3-945954-25-6

# Program

# 1$^{st}$ Symposium on Functional Autoantibodies Targeting G-Protein-Coupled Receptors

## 7 – 9 October 2016; Venue: Radisson Blu Senator Hotel, Lübeck

| Friday, 07.10.2016 | |
|---|---|
| | |
| 3:00pm - 8:00pm | Registration |
| 5:00pm - 5:20pm | **Welcome from the University President:** Hendrik Lehnert<br>**Welcome the Chair of the Symposium:** Gabriela Riemekasten |
| 5:20pm - 6:00pm | **Opening Lecture:** Autoantibodies against GPCR – a new principle to understand diseases |
| 6:00pm - 8:00pm | Welcome Reception |

| Saturday, 08.10.2016 | |
|---|---|
| | |
| 9:00am - 10:00am | **GPCRs and their modulation in neurological diseases**<br><br>**Madlen Löbel:** Immunoadsorption to remove ß adrenergic and M acetylcholine receptor antibodies in Chronic Fatigue Syndrome<br><br>**Lasse Melvaer Giil:** Antibodies to signaling molecules and receptors in Alzheimer's disease - Immune-related cognitive dysfunction and mortality.<br><br>**Oral presentations from selected abstracts** |
| 10:00am - 10:30am | Coffee break |
| 10:30am - 12:00pm | **GPCRs and their modulation in cardiovascular diseases**<br><br>**Florian Herse:** AT1-Autoantibodies in hypertensive disease of pregnancy<br><br>**Fritz Boege:** Agonistic autoantibodies against β1-adrenergic receptors in dilated cardiomyopathy |

| | |
|---|---|
| | **Annekathrin Haberland:** BC 007, an aptamer for the neutralization of functional autoantibodies directed against GPCR that are identified by a functional test<br><br>**Oral presentations from selected abstracts** |
| 12:00pm - 1:15pm | Lunch |
| 1:15pm - 2:00pm | Poster Session |
| 2:00pm - 3:00pm | **GPCRs and their modulation in hemato-oncological diseases**<br><br>**Thomas Luft** : Role of autoantibodies directed against GPCRs in GVHD after allogenic SCT<br><br>**Frank Gieseler:** PAR2, a G-protein coupled receptor protein (GPR11): Possible relevance of aberrant expression by tumor cells<br><br>**Oral presentations from selected abstracts** |
| 3:00pm - 3:30pm | Coffee Break |
| 3:30pm – 5:00pm | **GPCRs and their modulation in rheumatic diseases**<br><br>**Gabriela Riemekasten:** Antibodies against GPCR in systemic sclerosis<br><br>**Xinhua Yu:** Autoantibodies against peptides of GPCRs in primary Sjögren's syndrome<br><br>**Otávio Cabral-Marques:** Physiological IgG autoantibodies regulate a network of G protein coupled receptors and growth factors<br><br>**Oral presentations from selected abstracts** |
| 6:00pm - 8:00pm | Social event |
| 8:00pm | **Dinner at the "Kartoffelkeller" in the historical center of Lübeck** |

| Sunday, 08.10.2016 | |
|---|---|
| | |
| 9:00am – 10:30am | **GPCR antibodies and their signaling**<br><br>**Duska Dragun:** Personalized medicine for transplant recipients according to anti-GPCR antibody status<br><br>**Aurélie Philippe:** New approaches to study functional selectivity in GPCR signaling<br><br>**Christian Sadik:** SSc- IgG effects are mediated through distinct pathways in THP-1 cells<br><br>**Oral presentations from selected abstracts** |
| 10:30am - 11:00am | Coffee break |
| 11:00pm - 12:00am | **Therapeutic approaches regarding GPCR modulation**<br><br>**Roland Jahns:** Novel therapeutic approaches in cardiac autoimmunity: Blocking peptides against beta1-adrenoceptor autoantibodies<br><br>**Manuela Camino**: Autoantibodies against beta 1 adrenergic receptors in dilated cardiomiopathy in children - treatment with immunoadsorption<br><br>**Oral presentations from selected abstracts** |
| 12:00pm - 12:45am | **Panel discussion and closing remarks:** Gabriela Riemekasten<br>Future directions and therapeutic approaches |
| 12:45pm | Lunch |

# TABLE OF CONTENTS

# Session 1

# GPCRs and their modulation in neurological diseases

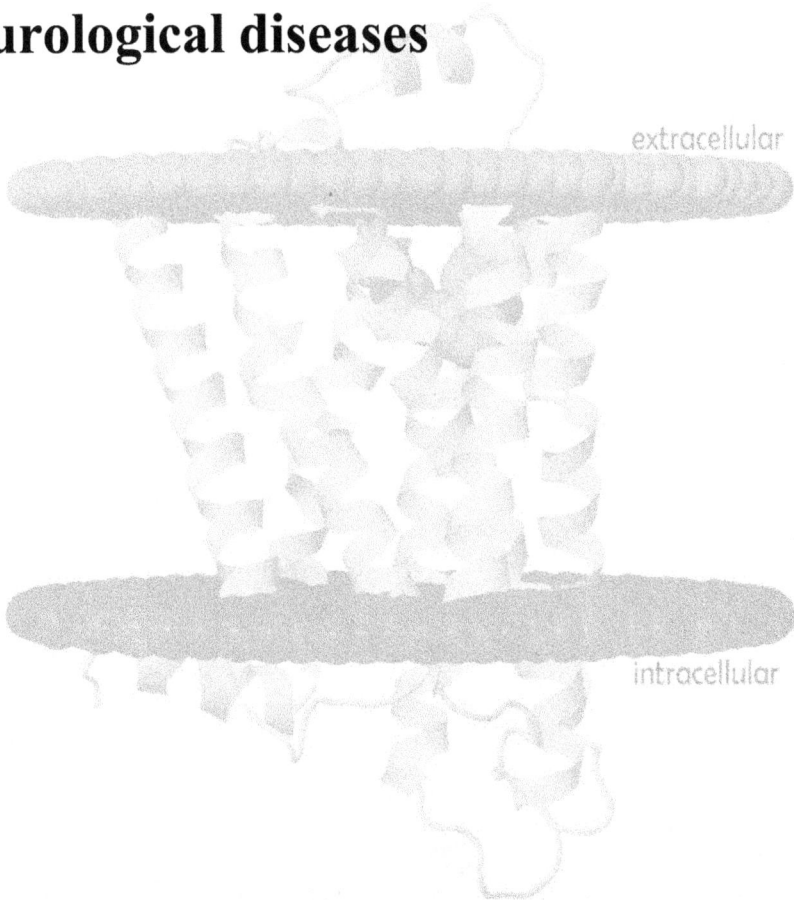

extracellular

intracellular

# Immunoadsorption to remove ß adrenergic and M acetylcholine receptor antibodies in Chronic Fatigue Syndrome

Madlen Loebel*[1], Patricia Grabowski[1], Harald Heidecke[2], Sandra Bauer[1], Michaela Antelmann[1], Anne Krueger[3], Petra Reinke[3,4], Wolfram Doehner[5], Hans-Dieter Volk[1,4], Carmen Scheibenbogen[1,4]

[1]*Institute for Medical Immunology, Charité Universitätsmedizin Berlin, Germany;* [2]*CellTrend GmbH, Luckenwalde, Germany;* [3]*Department of Nephrology, Charité Universitätsmedizin Berlin, Germany;* [4]*Berlin-Brandenburg Center for Regenerative Therapies (BCRT), Charité Universitätsmedizin Berlin, Germany;* [5]*Center for Stroke Research Berlin, Charité Universitätsmedizin Berlin, Germany.*

**Introduction.** Infection-triggered disease onset, chronic immune activation and autonomic dysregulation in CFS point to an autoimmune disease directed against neurotransmitter receptors. We could find elevated autoantibodies against ß2 adrenergic, and muscarinic (M) 3 and 4 acetylcholine receptors in a subset of patients (Löbel et al. 2016). Immunoadsorption (IA) was shown to be effective in removing autoantibodies against GPCRs and improve outcome in various autoimmune diseases.
**Methods.** 10 CFS patients with elevated ß2 adrenergic, some also with M 3/4 acetylcholine receptor antibodies were treated with an IgG-binding IA (Globaffin®) on 5 consecutive days with 2 – 2.5 fold of plasma volume filtered each day. We analysed total IgG and autoantibodies by ELISA in serum and characterized peripheral blood B cell phenotypes by flow cytometry.
**Results** Antibodies against ß2 adrenergic receptor were elevated in all CFS patients compared to the 90% percentile (8.45 U/ml) of a control group (n=108) prior to IA (CFS patients median 27.4, range 9.0-87.8 U/ml). In 9 of 10 patients ß2 antibodies rapidly decreased during IA to levels at or below 90% percentile of the control group. Similarly IgG decreased in all patients from median 10.89 g/l to 0.5 g/l after the last IA. Elevated M3 and M4 acetylcholine receptor antibodies were observed in a subset of patients and decreased in a similar manner. IgA and IgM levels remained unchanged. In the IA eluate high levels of ß2 autoantibodies were detected after the 1st IA. Comprehensive B cell typing was performed showing alterations in class-switched memory B cells and plasmablasts.
**Conclusion.** Autoantibodies against ß adrenergic and M acetylcholine receptors can be effectively removed by IA. IA was well tolerated and several patients reported rapid improvement of symptoms.

# Antibodies to signaling molecules and receptors in Alzheimer's disease - Immune-related cognitive dysfunction and mortality

Lasse Melvaer Giil

*Haraldsplass Deaconess University College, Internal medicine, Bergen, Norway*

Psychomotor speed, depression and visuospatial functions have been linked to peripheral immune activation as measured by serum and plasma levels of interleukin-6, 10 and CRP. The constellation of psychomotor speed reduction and depression has been called immune-related cognitive dysfunction, in the setting of increased inflammatory markers.

In our study on Alzheimer's disease, we see a strong relationship with several antibodies, in particular $D_1R$-ab, with trail making A, a test of psychomotor speed that is linked to excessive mortality. We also find that levels of ETAR-ab are linked to mild-to-moderate depression as measured by the Montgomery-Aasberg Depression Rating Scale (MADRS) and visuospatial function, measured by the Visual Object and Space Perception Battery (VOSP) to $HT_{1A}R$-ab. Furthermore, we find in AD that the effect depression has on psychomotor slowing can be explained by the association of depression with an interaction between antibodies and C-reactive protein (moderated mediation), suggesting that effects of of depression on psychomotor slowing is strongly related to immunological mechanisms.

Furthermore, there is a clear effect of antibodies on long-term mortality over a median survival time of 7.1 years, taking into account the effects of age, gender, psychomotor speed, depression and body-mass-index. The effect of the first principal component loaded by dopaminergic and serotonergic antibodies mainly, gave a hazard ratio of 2.84 (p = 0.001) in 90 patients with AD (68 censored cases) cross-validatet by bootstrap and jackknife estimates.

The antibodies with the clearest predictions for mortality were no different than in controls. This suggest that physiological antibodies perform physiological housekeeping functions, possibly linked to apoptosis and inflammation and less known housekeeping functions such as immune regulation or interactions with signaling systems. If they do in general have functional activity, potential drug-antibody interactions could become highly relevant, a topic under investigation by investigating drug-antibody interactions in statistical models from biobanks on heart failure and dementia. To further understand the role of physiological antibodies and the mechanism underpinning their association with mortality in AD, there is a need for epitope-mapping and development of standardized, functional immune-assays. This will strengthen the biological interpretation in large biomarker studies, particularly on longitudinal data. Experimental studies research on effects on the immune system and interactions with commonly prescribed medications that act on GPCRs would also be highly informative and hypothesis-generating.

# Session 2

# GPCRs and their modulation in cardiovascular diseases

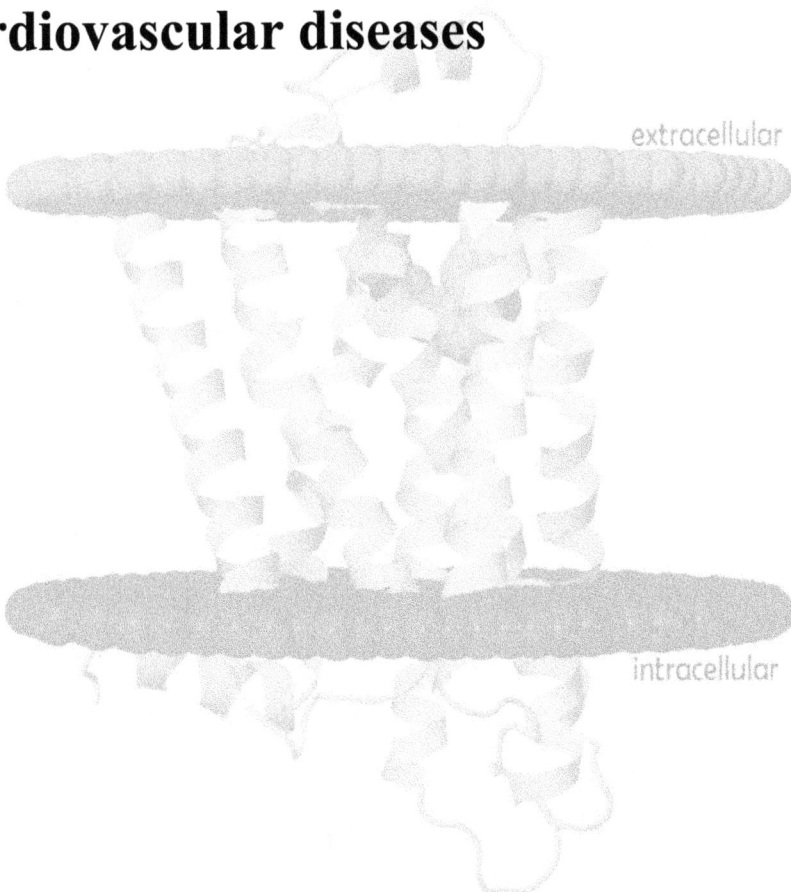

extracellular

intracellular

# AT1-Autoantibodies in hypertensive disease of pregnancy

Ralf Dechend[1,2,4], Florian Herse[1,2,3]

*[1]Experimental and Clinical Research Center, a joint cooperation between the Max-Delbrück Center for Molecular Medicine in the Helmholtz Association and the Charité Medical Faculty, Berlin, Germany; [2]Berlin Institute of Health (BIH), Berlin, Germany; [3]Max-Delbrück Center for Molecular Medicine in the Helmholtz Association, Berlin, German; [4]HELIOS-Klinikum, Berlin, Germany*

Autoantibodies can cause complications in pregnancy. Preeclampsia is a common, pregnancy- induced disorder, consisting of hypertension and proteinuria. The condition is one of the leading causes for maternal and perinatal morbidity and mortality and 5-10% of all pregnancies worldwide develop preeclampsia. Nonetheless, the underlying molecular mechanisms remain unclear. Immunological mechanisms and the renin-angiotensin system have been implicated in the development of preeclampsia. Agonistic autoantibodies to the angiotensin II type I receptor (AT1-AA) have been identified in preeclamptic patients. They induce NADPH oxidase and the MAPK/ERK pathway leading to NF-κB and tissue factor activation. AT1-AA are detectable in animal models of preeclampsia and are responsible for elevation of anti-angiogenic factors, oxidative stress and endothelin-1, all of which are enhanced in preeclamptic women. AT1-AA can be detected in pregnancies with abnormal uterine perfusion and increased resistance index as well as in patients with systemic sclerosis and renal allograft rejection.

# Agonistic autoantibodies against β1-andrenergic receptors in dilated cardiomyopathy

Fritz Boege

*Institute of Clinical Chemistry and Laboratory Diagnostics, University Hospital, Düsseldorf, Germany*

Autoantibodies against cardiac $\beta_1$-adrenergic receptors ($\beta_1$AR) cause or promote chronic heart failure (CHF) in the context of several aetiologies [1]. The cardio-noxious action of $\beta_1$AR-autoantibodies involves receptor activation and interference with receptor cycling [2]. The autoantibodies induce/stabilise an active conformation of the $\beta_1$AR-molecule [2] and fail to bind to chemically denatured $\beta_1$AR or peptide mimics thereof, which suggests that they target a conformational epitope associated with the activation state of the receptor. Epitope presentation is strongly biased by the common genetic $\beta_1$AR$^{389Gly/Ser}$ -polymorphism, which possibly confounds diagnostic determinations while not influencing the risk of chronic heart failure associated with receptor-autoimmunity [3].

Patients suffering from CHF due to β1AR autoimmunity could benefit from specific therapies, if potentially cardio-noxious β1AR autoantibodies were reliably diagnosed. Since the conformational epitope presumed CHF-relevant is inadequately presented by denatured β1AR or linear peptide mimics [1, 4, 5, 6, 7, 8], reliable diagnostic of CHF-relevant $\beta_1$AR autoantibodies so far requires assessment of functional effects or IgG-binding to native, cell-bound β1AR [7]. However, such tests are impractical for routine diagnostics. In consequence, currently, uncertainty about valid and practical procedures for the diagnostic determination of β1AR-autoantibodies delays the implementation of personalised, specific therapeutic approaches that are in principle available [9, 10, 11, 12, 13, 14, 15, 16, 17].

Recently, a binding assay for β1AR-autoantibodies has become commercially available, which allows a quantitative determination of the binding of serum IgG to native membranes from cell lines overexpressing the human β1AR. We have validated this CE-certified test using reference antibodies, reference methods and established cohorts of DCM-patients and healthy individuals with confirmed autoantibody status [2, 6, 7]. We come to the conclusion that the new diagnostic test provides a valid and versatile tool for quantitative diagnostic determinations of disease-relevant β1AR autoantibodies and may be useful as companion diagnostic for therapies specifically targeting β1AR autoantibodies in chronic heart failure.

References:

1. Bornholz B, Roggenbuck D, Jahns R, Boege F. Diagnostic and therapeutic aspects of beta-adrenergic receptor autoantibodies in human heart disease. *Autoimmun Rev* **13**, 954-962 (2014).
2. Bornholz B, *et al.* Impact of human autoantibodies on beta1-adrenergic receptor conformation, activity, and internalization. *Cardiovasc Res* **97**, 472-480 (2013).
3. Bornholz B, Hanzen B, Reinke Y, Felix SB, Boege F. Impact of common beta-adrenergic receptor polymorphisms on the interaction with agonistic autoantibodies in dilated cardiomyopathy. *Int J Cardiol* **214**, 83-85 (2016).
4. Jahns R, Boivin V, Siegmund C, Inselmann G, Lohse MJ, Boege F. Autoantibodies activating human beta1-adrenergic receptors are associated with reduced cardiac function in chronic heart failure. *Circulation* **99**, 649-654 (1999).
5. Jahns R, Boivin V, Krapf T, Wallukat G, Boege F, Lohse MJ. Modulation of beta(1)-adrenoceptor activity by domain-specific antibodies and-heart failure-associated autoantibodies. *J Am Coll Cardiol* **36**, 1280-1287 (2000).
6. Bornholz B, *et al.* A standardised FACS assay based on native, receptor transfected cells for the clinical diagnosis and monitoring of beta1-adrenergic receptor autoantibodies in human heart disease. *Clin Chem Lab Med* **54**, 683-691 (2016).
7. Bornholz B, *et al.* Detection of DCM-associated beta1-adrenergic receptor autoantibodies requires functional readouts or native human beta1-receptors as targets. *Int J Cardiol* **202**, 728-730 (2016).
8. Jahns R, Boege F. Questionable validity of petide-based ELISA strategies in the diagnostics of cadrdiopathogenic autoantibodies that activate G-protein-coupled receptors. *Cardiology* **131**, 149-150 (2015).
9. Munch G, *et al.* Administration of the cyclic peptide COR-1 in humans (phase I study): ex vivo measurements of anti-beta1-adrenergic receptor antibody neutralization and of immune parameters. *Eur J Heart Fail* **14**, 1230-1239 (2012).
10. Haberland A, *et al.* Neutralization of pathogenic beta1-receptor autoantibodies by aptamers in vivo: the first successful proof of principle in spontaneously hypertensive rats. *Molecular and cellular biochemistry* **393**, 177-180 (2014).
11. Haberland A, Wallukat G, Schimke I. Aptamer binding and neutralization of beta1-adrenoceptor autoantibodies: basics and a vision of its future in cardiomyopathy treatment. *Trends Cardiovasc Med* **21**, 177-182 (2011).
12. Haberland A, Wallukat G, Dahmen C, Kage A, Schimke I. Aptamer neutralization of beta1-adrenoceptor autoantibodies isolated from patients with cardiomyopathies. *Circulation research* **109**, 986-992 (2011).
13. Dandel M, *et al.* Immunoadsorption can improve cardiac function in transplant candidates with non-ischemic dilated cardiomyopathy associated with diabetes mellitus. *Atherosclerosis Supplements* **18**, 124-133 (2015).
14. Patel PA, Hernandez AF. Targeting anti-beta-1-adrenergic receptor antibodies for dilated cardiomyopathy. *Eur J Heart Fail* **15**, 724-729 (2013).
15. Boivin V, *et al.* Novel Receptor-Derived Cyclopeptides to Treat Heart Failure Caused by Anti-beta1-Adrenoceptor Antibodies in a Human-Analogous Rat Model. *PLoS One* **10**, e0117589 (2015).
16. Felix SB, *et al.* Removal of cardiodepressant antibodies in dilated cardiomyopathy by immunoadsorption. *J Am Coll Cardiol* **39**, 646-652 (2002).
17. Nnane IP, *et al.* Pharmacokinetics and Safety of Single Intravenous Doses of JNJ-54452840, an Anti-beta1-Adrenergic Receptor Antibody Cyclopeptide, in Healthy Male Japanese and Caucasian Participants. *Clinical pharmacokinetics* **55**, 225-236 (2016).

# BC 007, an aptamer for the neutralization of functional autoantibodies directed against GPCR that are identified by a functional test

Annekathrin Haberland[1] Ingolf Schimke[1], Katrin Wenzel[1], Niels-Peter Becker[1], Sarah Schulze-Rothe[1], Hanna Davideit[1], Susanne Becker[1], Peter Göttel[1], Gerd Wallukat[1], Johannes Müller*[1]

[1]Berlin Cures GmbH Berlin, Germany

**Introduction.** Aptamers, also called chemical antibodies, are able to bind to their targets with high affinity and have already been shown to efficiently neutralize functional activity of their target proteins even under *in-vivo* conditions. This also holds true for targeted autoantibodies (AAB). With BC 007 one aptamer was identified which is able to neutralize all pathogenic AABs tested so far which are directed to G-protein-coupled receptors.

**Methods.** The efficiency of BC 007 to neutralize G-protein-coupled receptor-AABs has been shown using the bioassay of spontaneously beating rat cardiomyocytes which excellently identifies the functional active AABs.

**Results.** Using the bioassay, it was shown that BC 007 neutralized the functional activity of AABs directed at the adrenergic alpha1-, beta2-, and beta1-receptor (specific for the 1st and 2nd extracellular loop of the receptor), the muscarinic M2-receptor, the PAR-, ETA1-, and AT1-receptors and others when incubated with autoantibodies. The addition of BC 007 after the AABs have already developed their full functional activity also led to a complete neutralization of the AAB-activity, a prerequisite for the *in-vivo* application. *In-vivo* BC 007 efficiently neutralized the AABs in beta1-AAB positive tested spontaneously hypertensive rats (SHR-rats). The beta1-AABs did not reoccur during the post-observation time of almost 100 days after treatment.

**Conclusion.** BC 007, a broad-spectrum neutralizer of the functional activity of G-protein-coupled receptor-AABs could be a breakthrough in the future treatment of diseases which are accompanied by the occurrence of pathogenic G-protein-coupled receptor-AABs such as dilated cardiomyopathy. Here the AAB-removal via immunoadsorption has already proven its enormous beneficial effect for the patients. The complex immunoadsorption therapy should be replaced by BC 007 application. BC 007 is currently in phase I of clinical testing.

# Agonistic autoantibodies as vascular damaging component in diabetes and dementia

Marion Bimmler*, Peter Karczewski, Bernd Lemke, Petra Hempel

*E.R.D.E.-AAK-Diagnostik GmbH Berlin, Germany*

**Introduction:** Agonistic acting autoantibodies (agAAB) occupy a special position among the autoantibodies. They bind to G-protein coupled receptors and act similar to the natural agonist. AgAAB do not respond to immunosupressiva, but can be removed from the receptor by their respective specific antagonists. The agAAB against the alpha-1 AR activate so important signaling molecules such as protein kinase C, induce the phosphorylation and thus a change in functionality of regulatory proteins in cardiac calcium homeostasis and influence the gene expression of the L-type calcium channel. The non-physiological and long-lasting activation of cellular processes caused by the action of agAAB, leads to the formation of pathological conditions such as calcium overload of the cell, remodeling of cell structures and even cell death, due to the long-lasting transformation of ATP into cAMP. In addition, they induce the proliferation of vascular smooth muscle cells. The result is a non-physiological thickening of the vessel wall with reduction of vessel lumen.

**Methods:** Presence and function of the various agAAB was tested in 3 independent test systems: peptide-based ELISA, cloned cell lines and bioassay.

**Result:** We could show, that 70% of patients with diabetes type 2, who are ill for more than 20 years, harbouring agAAB against the alpha-1-adrenergic receptor (AR), angiotensin receptor, beta-1-AR and/or endothelin A receptor (ETANoteworthy, agAAB against the alpha-1-AR can be detected in all diabetic patients who have suffered a heart attack or stroke. In patients with coronary heart disease, the prevalence was 91% of this agAAB.

In patients with dementia (Alzheimer's/vascular dementia) we found agAAB against the alpha-1-AR, beta-2-AR in 50% of patients. Removal of agAAB by immunoadsorption leads to stabilization in memory performance over a period of more than 18 months.

**Conclusion:** We suggest that this agAAB play (in part) an important role, why diabetics significantly more likely to suffer from dementia than people without diabetes.

# Session 3

# GPCRs and their modulation in hemato-oncological diseases

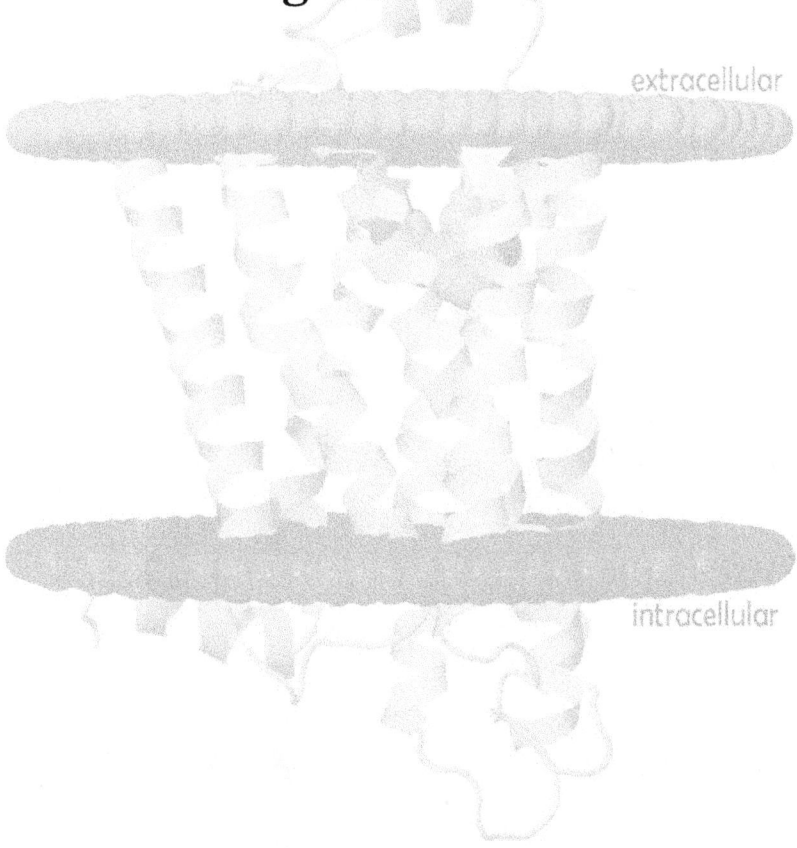

extracellular

intracellular

# Role of autoantibodies directed against GPCRs in graft-versus-host disease after allogenic stem cell transplantation

Thomas Luft

*University Hospital Heidelberg, Dept. of Medicine V*

Allogeneic stem cell transplantation (alloSCT) is a curative treatment option for patients suffering from leukemia and other hematological malignancies. Acute graft-versus-host disease (GVHD) frequently occurs after alloSCT and is primarily treated with corticosteroids. If steroid treatment fails - a condition termed refractory GVHD (refrGVHD) – mortality is very high without considerable improvement during the last decades. Currently there is no standard procedure for prediction of GVHD-related mortality at onset of GVHD, impeding the implementation of risk adapted GVHD treatment approaches in clinical practice.

There is a growing body of evidence that endothelial damage contributes to refractoriness of GVHD. Our group has reported markers of endothelial vulnerability that are predictive of steroid refractoriness such as angiopoietin-2, soluble thrombomodulin, serum nitrates and assymetric di-methyl-arginine (ADMA). Furthermore, genetic variants within the recipient's thrombomodulin (THBD) gene also predict mortality of manifest GVHD. However, the nature of the endothelial cell problem associated with refractoriness of acute GVHD remains unspecified.

As G-Protein-coupled receptors are expressed on the surface of endothelial cells, we hypothesized that autoantibodies targeting these receptors might modulate the outcome of endothelial complications after allogeneic stem cell transplantation.

We will report how auto-antibodies against GPCR associate with outcome of patients with GVHD.

# PAR2, a G-protein coupled receptor protein (GPR11): Possible relevance of aberrant expression by tumor cells

Corinna Plattfaut, Annika Freund, Christian Haas, Frank Gieseler*

*UKSH Campus Luebeck, University Hospital and Medical School, Luebeck, Germany*

Protease activated receptors (PARs) are integral membrane proteins that are coupled to G-proteins. Four types of PARs have been identified. They are activated by specific cleavage of the amino terminal sequence that exposes an N-terminal sequence. This functions as a tethered ligand that binds intra-molecularly to activate the receptor.

In contrast to the other members of the PAR family, which are activated by the protease thrombin, PAR2 is activated by trypsin and tissue-factor complexes that are formed during activation of the extrinsic pathway of the coagulation system. The coagulation system is regularly activated in inflammatory conditions and during cancer progression and metastasis, resulting in venous thrombotic events a major reason for both morbidity and mortality.

In 1991 Coughlin isolated the encoding sequence of PAR1, located on thrombocytes. The main activating protease is thrombin. Others and we have shown that PAR1 is aberrantly expressed on most tumor cells from different origins. PAR2 was detected in 1994 in a mouse genomic library, due to its high similarity with the human PAR1 receptor. Mostly, PAR1 and PAR2 are co-expressed on cancer cells.

Various cells including tumor cells release tissue factor bearing extracellular vesicles (EVs) during inflammatory processes. We have shown that PAR2 located on tumor cells is activated by these EVs. Several intracellular pathways triggered by PAR2 have been described. They involve interactions at membrane level, e.g. functional interaction of PAR2 with TGFbeta, cytosolic effects, e.g. binding to beta-arrestin as chaperon, and ERK1/2 phosphorylation. The latter is associated with EMT of tumor cells and the induction of migration - a significant surrogate parameter for tumor progression and metastasis.

We isolated tissue factor bearing EVs from several patient sources such as peripheral blood, malignant effusions and urine and identified molecular parameters decisive for PAR2 stimulation, the G-protein pathway-activation and tumor cell migration as cellular answer.

These observations establish a link between inflammation, activation of the coagulation system and cancer progression. Diagnostic and therapeutic consequences such as the use of GPR antibodies can be discussed.

# Session 4

# GPCRs and their modulation in rheumatic diseases

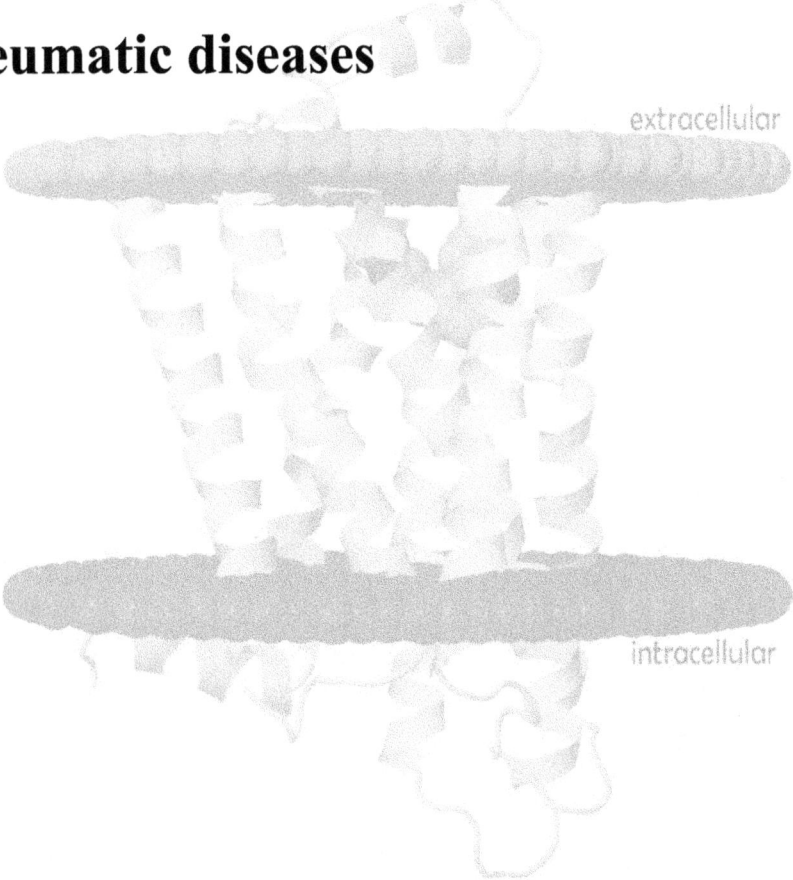

extracellular

intracellular

# Functional autoantibodies against GPCR in systemic sclerosis

Gabriela Riemekasten[1], Judith Rademacher[2,3], Jeannine Günther[2,3], Angela Kill[2,3], Otavio Cabral-Marques[1]

[1]Dept. of Rheumatology, University of Lübeck, Lübeck, Germany; [2]Dept. of Rheumatology and Clinical Immunology, Charité University Hospital, Berlin, Germany; [3]Cell Autoimmunity, DRFZ, Berlin, Germany

Systemic sclerosis is a systemic autoimmune disease with obliterative vasculopathy and fibrosis. Increased concentrations of autoantibodies against angiotensin receptor type 1 (AT1R) and endothelin receptor type-A (ETAR) are present in the majority of SSc patients. Both antibodies strongly correlate with each other's. The antibodies are associated with clinical symptoms such as PAH, lung fibrosis, digital ulcers, and renal crisis. High concentrations predict mortality, the incidence of new digital ulcers, and of PAH; low concentrations predict better response to therapies. In addition, receptor expressions of AT1R and ETAR on immune cells such as monocytes are increased, especially in early disease and linked with some clinical symptoms. The ratios of AT1R/AT2R and ETAR/ETBR are different compared to the corresponding ratios in healthy donors. In the last few years, we have studied the functional role of the antibodies against AT1R and ETAR. IgG from SSc patients induced signs of interstitial lung disease and vasculopathy in mice indicating a pathogenic role of antibodies. In addition, we have performed many in vitro experiments and have used the corresponding receptor blockers to identify functional effects on immune cells, endothelial cells, and fibroblasts. Several mechanisms known to be important in systemic sclerosis have been recognized as mediated by ETAR and AT1R. Nevertheless, not all effects were ameliorated by these blockers. In addition, we have studied other antibodies against GPCR and have identified several anti-GPCR antibodies either increased or decreased in SSc. Among them, anti-CXCR3 and anti-CXCR4 antibodies are increased in patients with SSc, too. However; high levels predict a milder form of SSc, particularly of lung fibrosis. Hierarchical cluster analyses of several autoantibodies present in SSc show high correlations of autoantibodies and certain patterns of antibodies, which strongly correlate with each other's. Taken together, systemic sclerosis seems to be a very interesting disease to study anti-GPCR antibodies. High antibody concentrations against AT1R and ETAR, increased receptor expression, and increased concentrations of the natural ligand make this disease as a prototypic disease for anti-AT1R/ETAR autoantibodies. Nevertheless, some other autoantibodies seem to modulate the effects of these antibodies. In the future, we hope to link antibody patterns with the clinical phenotype in SSc.

# Autoantibodies against peptides of GPCRs in primary Sjögren's syndrome

Xinhua Yu[1,2*]

[1]Research Center Borstel, Borstel, Germany and
[2]Xiamen-Borstel Joint Laboratory of Autoimmunity, Xiamen University, China

**Introduction.** Autoantibodies against GPCR, e.g. muscarinic acetylcholine type-3 receptor (M3R) are believe to play an important role in the pathogenesis of primary Sjögren's syndrome (pSS), and the second extracellular loop (2ndEL) of M3R is suspected to carry adisease-promoting epitope. Here we investigated the autoantibodies against the peptides of the extracellular domain of GPCR in pSS.

**Methods.** The profile of autoantibodies against the peptides of the extracellular domains of 25 GPCRs were determined by using a peptide microarray. Autoantibodies against the the second extracellular loop (2ndEL) of M3R was determined by using a peptide-based ELISA. Mice were immunized with peptides of the 2ndEL of M3R using CFA as adjuvant. The function of exocrine glands was evaluated by measuring the secretion of saliva and tears. The histological evaluations were performed by using H&E staining or direct immunofluorescence staining.

**Results.** Interestingly, SSA+ pSS patients differ significantly from SSA- pSS patients in the profiles of autoantibodie against peptides of GPCRs, with higher levels of those autoantibodies in SSA- pSS patients than in SSA+ patients. Using a peptide-based ELISA, our study shows that the prevalence of autoantibodies against the 2ndEL of M3R is low in pSS patients and it does not differ significantly from that in healthy controls. Furthermore, mice immunized with the peptides of the 2ndEL of M3R mice generated the peptide-specific autoantibodies which show week tissue binding activity. However, no significant difference in tears and saliva secretion was observed between immunized mice and controls, suggesting no dysfunction of exocrine glands.

**Conclusion.** Our results suggest that the autoantibodies against peptides of the second extracellular loop of M3R are not pathogenic *in vivo* and they are not suitable as biomarkers for pSS diagnosis.

# Physiological IgG autoantibodies regulate a network of G protein coupled receptors and growth factors

Otavio Cabral-Marques[a], Antje Mueller[a], Silke Pitann[a], Lasse Melvær Giil[d], Judith Rademacher[c,d], Jeannine Günther[c,d], Jing Sun[e], Anja Kerstein[a], Gabriele Marschner[a], Sabine Adler[f], Xinhua-Yu[g], Ralf Dechend[h,i], Dominik Müller[h,i], Duska Dragun[j], Ioana Braicu[j], Jalid Sehouli[l], Kai Schulze-Forster[m,n], Tobias Trippel[o], Carmen Scheibenbogen[p,q], Annetine Staff[s], Peter R. Mertens[t], Tanja Lange[a], Madlen Löbel[p], Jens Y Humrich[a], Christian D. Sadik[u], Harald Heidecke[n], Peter Lamprecht[a] and Gabriela Riemekasten[a,c,d]

[a]Dept. of Rheumatology, University of Lübeck, Lübeck, Germany; [b]Deaconess Hospital, University of Bergen, Bergen, Norway; [c]Dept. of Rheumatology and Clinical Immunology, Charité University Hospital, Berlin, Germany; [d]Cell Autoimmunity Group, German Rheumatism Research Center (DRFZ), Berlin, Germany; [e]University of Cincinnati College of Medicine; Cincinnati, Ohio, USA. [f]University Hospital and University of Bern, Bern, Switzerland; [g]Research Center Borstel, Airway Research Center North (ARCN), Members of the German Center for Lung Research (DZL), Borstel, Germany; [h]Max-Delbrueck Center for Molecular Medicine, Berlin and Charité University Hospital, Berlin, Germany; [i]Dept. of Cardiology and Nephrology, HELIOS-Klinikum Berlin, Berlin, Germany[j]Dept. of Nephrology and Cardiovascular Research, Campus Virchow, Charité University Hospital, Berlin, Germany; [l]Dept. of Gynecology, Charité University Hospital, Berlin and Tumor Bank Ovarian Cancer Network (TOC), Berlin, Germany; [m]Dept. of Urology, Charité University Hospital, Berlin, Germany; [n]CellTrend GmbH, Luckenwalde, Brandenburg, Germany; [o]Dept. of Internal Medicine&Cardiology, Charité University Hospital, Berlin, Germany. [p]Institute for Medical Immunology, Charité University Hospital Berlin, Campus Virchow, Berlin, Germany; [q]Berlin-Brandenburg Center for Regenerative Therapies (BCRT), Charité University Hospital Berlin, Germany; [s]Norwegian Knowledge Centre for the Health Services, Oslo, Norway; [t]Institution: University Clinic for Nephrology and Hypertension, Diabetology and Endocrinology, University Hospital Magdeburg; [u]Department of Dermatology, University of Lübeck, Lübeck, Germany.

The role of autoantibodies in physiology is under debate. By investigating autoantibody (ab) concentrations against G protein-coupled receptors (GPCR) in different autoimmune diseases we found both increased as well as decreased ab concentrations suggesting physiological anti-GPCR ab levels and their dysregulation in autoimmune diseases. Expansion of antibody analyses to 16 GPCR, 15 growth factors and related signaling molecules in healthy donors revealed clusters of correlations of antibody concentrations. Possible functional interactions of the 31 autoantibody target molecules were studied by STRING, DAVID, and enriched Gene Ontology analyses and revealed a network of GPCR, growth factors, and signaling molecules with endothelin receptor type A (ETAR) in the center. Migration and locomotion were suggested to be the most significant functions regulated by the antibody network. Accordingly, IgG from healthy donors induced both IL-8 expression by peripheral blood mononuclear cells (PBMCs) as well as migration of neutrophils, which was specifically diminished by the ETAR blocker sitaxentan. In conclusion, we identified that IgG autoantibodies physiologically regulate a GPCR and growth factor network for cell migration. In addition, our data indicate a novel approach to understand diseases and provide rationales for therapies.

# Session 5

# GPCR antibodies and their signaling

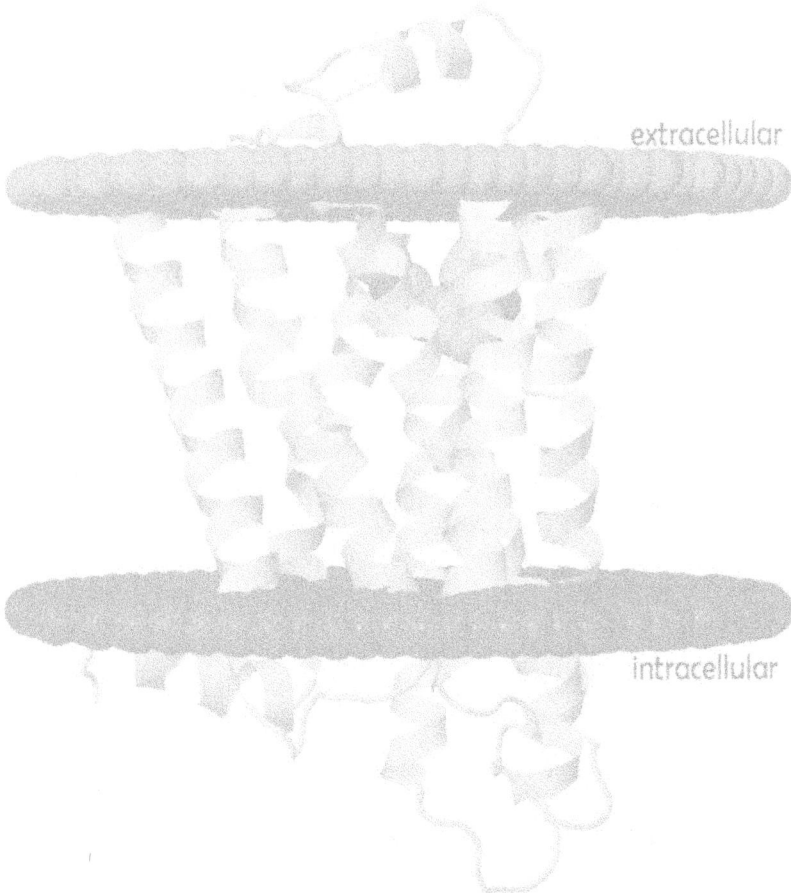

extracellular

intracellular

# Personalized medicine for transplant recipients according to anti-GPCR antibody status

Prof. Dr. Duska Dragun

*Medizinische Klinik mit Schwerpunkt Nephrologie und Internistische Intensivmedizin, Charité Universitätsmedizin Berlin, Berlin; Berliner Institut für Gesundheitsforschung, Berlin*

Detrimental actions of donor specific antibodies directed against both major histoincompatibility antigens (HLA-DSA) and specific non-HLA antigens expressed on the allograft endothelium are flourishing research area in all field of solid organ and stem cell transplantation. Newly developed solid-phase assays enabling detection of functional non-HLA antibodies targeting G-protein coupled receptors such as Angiotensin type 1 receptor (AT1R) and Endothelin type A receptor (ETAR) were instrumental in providing long-awaited confirmation for their broad clinical relevance. Numerous recent clinical studies implicate AT1R- and ETAR-antibodies as prognostic biomarkers for earlier occurrence and severity of acute and chronic immunologic complications in solid organ transplantation, stem cell transplantation, and systemic autoimmune vascular disease. AT1R- and ETAR-antibodies exert their pathophysiological effects alone and in synergy with HLA-DSA. Comprehensive diagnostic assessment strategies focusing on both HLA-DSA and AT1R- and ETAR-antibodies - non-HLA-antibody responses could substantially improve immunologic risk-stratification already before transplantation, help to better define subphenotypes of antibody-mediated rejection, and lead to timely initiation of targeted therapies. Better understanding of functional selectivity in pathways mediating endothelial damage should facilitate discovery of common targets and pave the way for development of endothelium-centered therapeutic strategies to accompany intensified immunosuppression and/or mechanical removal of antibodies.

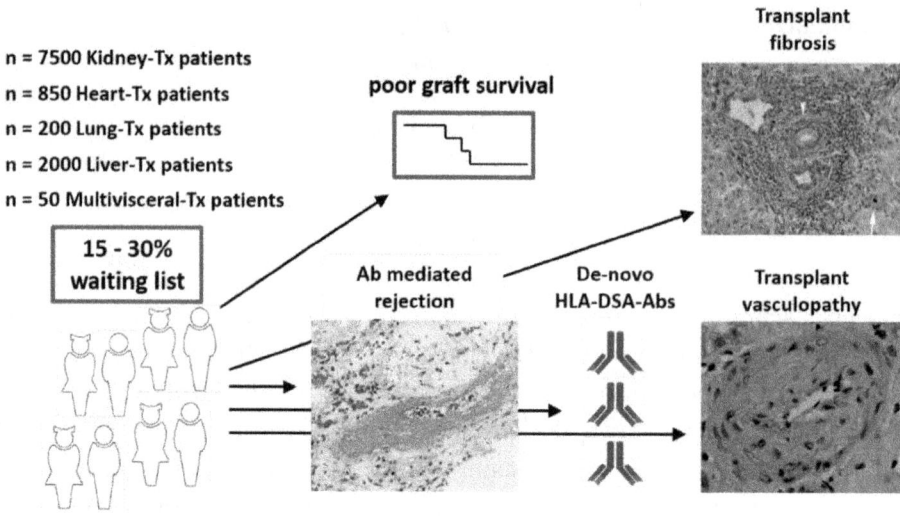

n = 7500 Kidney-Tx patients
n = 850 Heart-Tx patients
n = 200 Lung-Tx patients
n = 2000 Liver-Tx patients
n = 50 Multivisceral-Tx patients

15 - 30% waiting list

poor graft survival

Transplant fibrosis

Ab mediated rejection

De-novo HLA-DSA-Abs

Transplant vasculopathy

# New approaches to study functional selectivity in GPCR signaling

Philippe Aurélie

*AG Prof. Dragun, Medizinische Klinik mit Schwerpunkt Nephrologie und internistische Intensivmedizin, CVK, Charité Universitätsmedizin Berlin*

A wide range of untreatable or difficult to treat disease entities are caused by activating autoantibodies directed against G-protein coupled receptors (GPCR). Hence, molecular architecture of the binding of these antibodies to the receptors and the functional consequences of changes in specific structural modules are of immense clinical relevance not only for mechanistic understanding but even more important for later molecular drug design endeavours. Our laboratory has focused over the years on the Angiotensin II type 1 receptor ($AT_1R$), which exhibits multiligand binding abilities and signals upon endogenous Angiotensin II (Ang II)-mediated and $AT_1R$-agonistic IgG ($AT_1R$-Abs)-mediated stimulation. Development of high-resolution methods allows for structural-functional relationship studies of specific receptor modules, including the extracellular domains, in the receptor activation.

To distinguish the $AT_1R$ endogenous and immune-mediated activation, we first developed a yeast model where human GPCR activation controls yeasts growth. These yeasts have been modified to express one single human GPCR that couples to a chimera between human and yeast G-protein. Each yeast strain is specific of a different G-protein. Activation of the human GPCR with the appropriate stimulus triggers an intracellular signalling pathway mediated by ERK1/2 resulting in the growth of the yeasts.

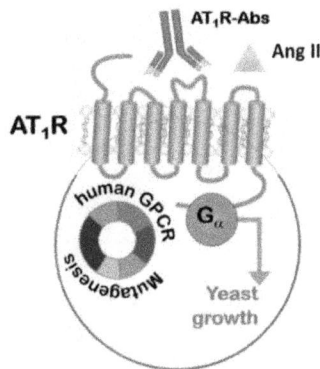

Validation of the model is performed using the endogenous peptide agonist of the receptor, Ang II, and $AT_1R$ blocker, Valsartan. Point mutations can be introduced by site-directed mutagenesis in order to determine the influence of amino acids sequences on the receptor activation. To investigate further the link between conformation and activation of the receptor in a more complicated environment, we performed luciferase reporter assays in Human Microvascular Endothelial Cells (HMEC-1) after transfecting the cells with wild type or mutated $AT_1$ receptor and the appropriate reporter plasmids. Comparison between wild type and mutants, non-stimulated and stimulated cells allowed us to better characterize the influence of the conformation changes on $AT_1R$ activation.

We successfully created models allowing for structural and functional studies of molecular architecture modules appreciating $AT_1R$ receptor plasticity, which helped us to define the role of the specific extracellular domains. Better understanding of the molecular mechanisms responsible for $AT_1R$ activation holds great potential for design of more specific AT1R blockers.

# SSc- IgG effects are mediated through distinct pathways in THP-1 cells

Georgios Eleftheriadis[1], Melanie Wannick[1], Christian Sadik[1]*, Gabriela Riemekasten[2]*

* CDS and GR contributed equally

[1]*Lübeck Institute of Experimental Dermatology, University of Lübeck, Lübeck, German;* [2]*Dept. of Rheumatology, University of Lübeck, Lübeck, Germany*

**Background**: Peripheral-blood-mononuclear-cells (PBMCs) are thought to play a key role in the pathogenesis and progress of systemic scleroderma (SSc) with patients displaying distinct shifts in count, receptor expression profile and cytokine secretion patterns. SSc-IgG with elevated anti-$AT_1R$ (angiotensin II type 1 receptor )/$ET_AR$ (endothelin-1 type A receptor) -AAb (autoantibody) titers has been correlated to disease severity and progression. It remains poorly understood through which pathways SSc- IgG mediates its effects.

**Aim**: In this study we sought to analyze the expression patterns of THP-1 cells (a monocytic cell line) after SSc-IgG application and their reversibility through application of numerous pharmacological inhibitors

**Methods**: Transcription of IL-8- and CCL-18 in THP-1-cells after SSc-IgG and normal IgG stimulation was quantified by qPCR. Stimulations of THP-1 cells with total IgG of phenotypically different groups of SSc-patients as well as ET-1 and AT-2 were carried out. In addition, stimulation with pharmacological inhibitors was conducted in a dose-dependent-manner. The results were quantified by IL-8- and CCL18-ELISA of the supernatants.

**Results**: Expression of IL-8 and CCL 18 is induced by SSc-IgG treatment in comparison to normal IgG which does not follow this trend. IL-8 secretion of THP-1 cells upon SSc-IgG stimulation is mediated through specific autoantibody effects and transduced through NF-κB, ERK-, and AP-1 pathways. CCL 18 secretion of THP-1 cells upon SSc-IgG stimulated is not mediated through aforementioned pathways.

**Conclusion**: A stable cell culture system able to reproduce previous PBMC data on IL-8 and CCL-18 induction upon SSc- IgG-treatment could be established and insight was gained regarding key pathways which are involved in the transduction leading to IL-8 secretion. The effects of specific surface receptor expression profiles on transduction remains to be elucidated.

# Galectin-3 binds highly galactosylated IgG1 and is crucial for the IgG1 complex mediated inhibition of GPCR induced immune responses

Kerstin A. Heyl[1], Hortense Slevogt[1], Christian M. Karsten[2*]

[1]*Septomics Research Center, Jena University Hospital, Jena, Germany; [2]Institute for Systemic Inflammation Research, University of Lübeck, Lübeck, Germany*

**Introduction**: Changes in the glycosylation of immunoglobulins have been shown to modulate immune homeostasis and disease pathology. In this sense it has been shown that highly galactosylated but not agalactosylated IgG1 immune complexes (ICs) inhibit GPCR-mediated pro-inflammatory immune responses via the assembly of FcγRIIB-Dectin-1 receptor complexes. In this study we show that Galectin-3, a galactose-binding lectin, which is known to cross-link proteins on cell-surfaces via binding their N-glycans, binds to highly-galactosylated, but not agalactosylated IgG1 ICs. Further, Galectin-3 was essential for the IC-mediated inhibition of C5a-induced neutrophil chemotaxis *in vitro*.

**Methods**: We used surface plasmon resonance (SPR) and immunoprecipitation (IP) assays to show differential binding of Galectin-3 to either high or low galactosylated IgG1 ICs. Further we tested the functional consequences of Galctin-3 binding to IgG1 ICs on C5a-induced chemotaxis of neutrophils.

**Results**: First we showed that the cells we used are able to express Galectin-3. For that reason, neutrophils were lysed by cellular factions and analyzed for Galectin-3 expression via Western Blot analysis. We detected Galectin-3 protein in the whole cell lysate, the cytosol and in the membrane fraction. Secondly we showed the binding of Galectin-3 to high but not to low galactosylated IgG1 ICs using SPR and IP assays. In a final test we confirmed using a modified boyden chamber that only in the presence of Galectin-3 high galactosylated IgG1 ICs are able to inhibit C5a-induced chemotaxis.

**Conclusion**: In this study we showed that binding of Galectin-3 to highly galactosylated IgG1 ICs compared to reduced binding to agalactosylated IgG1 ICs might serve as the missing link to explain the ability or inability of ICs to suppress GPCR-induced effector functions, depending on IgG1-galactosylation.

# Session 6

# Therapeutic approaches regarding GPCR modulation

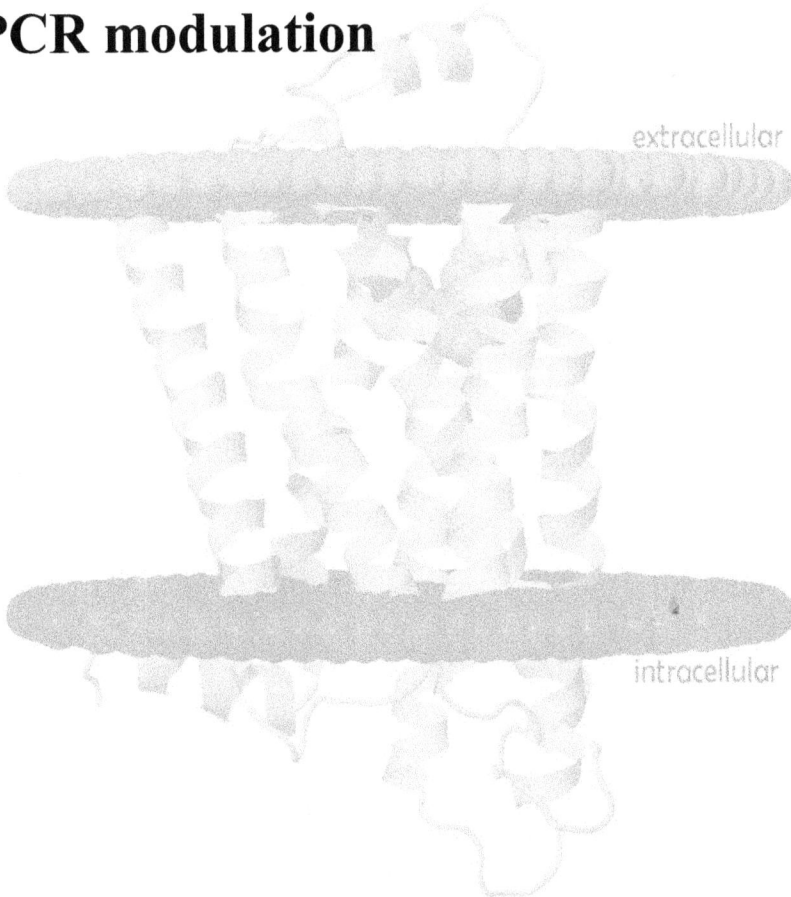

extracellular

intracellular

# Novel therapeutic approaches in cardiac autoimmunity: Blocking peptides against beta1-adrenoceptor autoantibodies

Roland Jahns

*Comprehensive Heart Failure Center (CHFC) and Interdisciplinary Bank of Biomaterials and Data (ibdw), University Hospital of Würzburg, Würzburg, Germany*

**Background and rationale**: Many cases of DCM are thought to arise from an acute or sub-acute myo-carditis which may progress to chronic auto-immune myocarditis resulting in cardiac dilatation and heart failure (HF), particularly, when associated (**a**) with the development of auto-antibodies against distinct myocyte or membrane proteins relevant for cardiac function, or (**b**) with chronic myocardial inflammation and virus persistence. Anti-beta1-adrenoceptor auto-antibodies (anti-beta1-abs) are thought to play a causal role in the pathogenesis of DCM; their prevalence (range: 26-60%) predicts poor prognosis.

Anti-beta1-abs that bind to and (chronically) stimulate the cardiac beta1-receptor are considered negative prognostic markers associated with a more severely reduced left ventricular function, an increase in serious ventricular arrhythmias and sudden cardiac death, and an about three-fold higher risk for cardiovascular death. Therefore, new therapeutic strategies that neutralize such auto-antibodies may provide a viable therapeutic strategy.

**Methods and results:** In this aim, recently, we have developed a cyclic peptide-mimic of the beta1-AR epitope supposed to be targeted by stimulating anti-beta1-abs, e.g., the second extra-cellular domain of the beta1-adrenergic receptor (beta1ECII, 100% sequence homology human/rat). It acts through scavenging of anti-beta1ECII-abs in the circulating blood directly after injection and decreases anti-beta1-specific memory-B cells producing anti-beta1ECII-abs without affecting overall B-cell count.

*Pre-clinical studies:* Stimulating anti-beta1ECII-abs cause dilated immune-cardiomyopathy in a human-analogous rat-model. In this model we tested the dose-dependent therapeutic efficacy of 4-weekly injections of ECII-CP on the development of heart failure (HF). Compared with untreated immunized rats after 6 and 12 injections of 0.3, 1.0, or 3.0 mg ECII-CP/kg/month anti-beta1-ECII-titers were reduced to 89%, 62% or 49%, and 76%, 46%, or 30% of the titres at start of therapy, respectively. However, regarding reversal of the DCM phenotype 1.0 mg ECII-CP/kg was clearly more efficient than either 0.3 or 3.0mg/kg doses, suggesting the existence of a stoichiometric optimum for anti-beta1-ab/ECII-CP-interactions.

*Clinical studies:* In pre-clinical studies 4-weekly injections of ECII-CP either prevented or treated anti-beta1-ab-induced myocardial damage in the rat along with an almost complete reversal of the cardiomyopathic phenotype. For clinical testing 4-weekly i.v.-applications of ECII-CP were planned as an add-on to HF-standard therapy. A phase I, placebo-controlled clinical study in healthy volunteers supported a good tolerability profile of ECII-CP. In anti-beta1-ab-spiked sera of phase-I study-participants, ECII-CP in a dose-dependent manner almost completely scavenged all anti-beta1-abs present in the samples. Half-life of ECII-CP was in the range of minutes, and clearance was rapid after i.v.- application. No neutralising anti-ECII-CP antibodies occurred in healthy volunteers.

Next, a double-blind pilot phase II-study was initiated to analyze the effects of 6 injections of ECII-CP every 4 weeks as add-on to standard HF therapy on cardiac function of HF patients with DCM. Eligible antibody-positive DCM patients received either placebo or ECII-CP (0.3, 1.0, or 3.0mg/kg administered intravenously every 4 weeks). Primary endpoint was the change in left ventricular ejection fraction (LVEF) from baseline to month 6 determined by biplane echocardiography. In this pilot-study an increase in LVEF (> 5%) compared to placebo was noted in the 1.0 mg/kg ECII-CP treated group only, along with a non-significant reduction in anti-beta1-ab titers.

**Conclusions:** Stimulating antibodies directed against the ECII-domain of the beta1-adrenoceptor (beta1ECII; 100% sequence homology rat/human) induce dilated immune-cardiomyopathy in rats. In this pre-clinical model, monthly injection of 1.0 mg/kg beta1ECII-homologous cyclic scavenger peptides (ECII-CP) reversed the cardiomyopathic phenotype. ECII-CP was well tolerated in a placebo-controlled clinical phase I-study in healthy volunteers. A subsequently initiated clinical phase-II pilot study suggests clinical efficacy of 1.0 mg/kg ECII-CP in antibody-positive DCM patients, but not at lower or higher doses. As in our rat model this suggests existence of a stoichiometric optimum for antibody/ECII-CP-interactions. However, another important limitation and/or pre-condition remaining to establish before broad clinical testing of ECII-CP is a reliable diagnostic tool for the determination of circulating functional anti-beta1-abs, which cannot be achieved by a simple peptide-ELISA requiring alternative detection strategies that turned out to be by far more difficult and complex in human patients than in immunized rats.

# BETA-1 Adrenergic-Receptor Antibodies in dilated Cardiomyopathy in Children and their Response to an Immunoadsorption Therapy

Manuela Camino MD

*Pediatric Heart Transplantation Unit, Gregorio Marañon Childrens Hospital, Madrid*

Over the past few decades, β1-adrenergic autoantibodies have been reported in sera from adult patients with dilated cardiomyopathy (DCM). The removal of these antibodies and/or its neutralization (blocking of the antibody-mediated action) have demonstrated a hemodynamic benefit and even the complete remission of the disease.

Our study aimed to determine the presence of β1-adrenergic autoantibodies in children with DCM as well as the potential hemodynamic benefit upon their removal by immunoadsorption (IA).

**Material and Methods:** We have tested the concentration of β1-adrenergic autoantibodies in 17 children (aged, 1-3 y.o.). The etiology of DCM was heterogeneous: genetics (n = 4), myocarditis (n = 3), mother lupus-associated congenital heart block (n = 3), and idiopathic (n = 7). All patients evidenced moderate-to-severe ventricle dysfunction and a left-ventricle ejection fraction (LVEF) lower than 50%, and NYHA II-IV. Serum samples were collected and sent to CellTrend facilities (Lukenwalde, Berlin) for each antibody determination (ELISA, positive if ≥15 U/ml). Immunoadsorption cycle therapy (4 session/cycle) was conducted in those patients with a positive testing to β1-adrenergic autoantibodies. Extracorporeal immunoadsorption was achieved with the TheraSorb Ig flex adsorbers (Miltenyi Biotec, GmbH).

**Results:** Antibody testing resulted to be positive in 7 patients (2 DCM, 2 idiopathic DCM, and 3 with myocarditis). All genetic-based cases were negative for the antibody determination.

IA therapy was done in 7 children. The tolerability of the technique was excellent, despite the hemodynamic compromise of these patients. BNP concentration was lowered after each IA cycle. Those patients (n = 3) who showed the highest concentration of autoantibodies (> 100 U/ml) also showed the poorest clinical outcome and they had to be heart-transplanted. Two patients with lower amounts of β1-adrenergic autoantibodies demonstrated a complete recovery of the heart function after just one cycle of IA. One patient died because of a sepsis after 15 months of follow-up, with an enhancement of his heart functional class and LEFV 45% though. Another patient showed a parvovirus-mediated myocarditis with a periodic rebound of the antibody levels that was treated with a combination of immunoglobulin iv (IVIG) and IA. Nowadays, and after 5 years of therapy, this patient evidences a NYHA-II and LVEF 45%.

**Conclusions:** β1-adrenergic autoantibodies are also circulating in the plasma of DCM children. The present finding may help identify the autoimmune mechanisms (myocarditis, lupus) of the heart failure. The evaluation of these antibodies will allow us to go for a better immunologic therapy (immunoglobulins, immunoadsorption) in order to associate this with other conventional treatment strategies to enhance or even reverse the condition of heart failure.

# Poster Abstracts

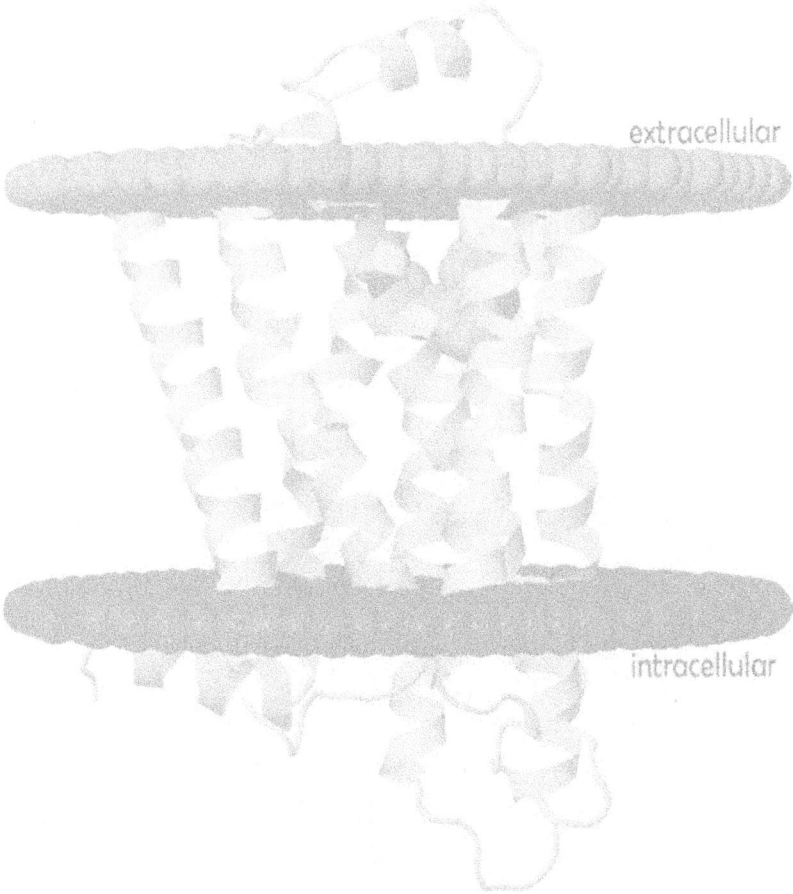

extracellular

intracellular

# Epinephrine suppresses integrin activity of stimulated cytomegalovirus-specific T cells in healthy humans

Tanja Lange*[1], Antje Müller[1], Luciana Besedovsky[2], Anja Tatiana Ramstedt Jensen[3], Jan Born[2,4,5,6], Cécile Gouttefangeas[7], Hans-Georg Rammensee[7], Gabriela Riemekasten[1], Stoyan Dimitrov[2,4,5]

[1]Department of Rheumatology, University of Lübeck, Lübeck, Germany, [2]Department of Medical Psychology and Behavioral Neurobiology, University of Tübingen, Tübingen, Germany. [3]Department of Immunology and Microbiology, University of Copenhagen, Copenhagen, Denmark. [4]Institute for Diabetes Research and Metabolic Diseases of the Helmholtz Center Munich at the University of Tübingen (IDM). [5]German Center for Diabetes Research (DZD), Tübingen, Germany. [6]Center for Integrative Neuroscience, University of Tübingen, Tübingen, Germany. [7]Department of Immunology, Institute for Cell Biology, University of Tübingen, Tübingen, Germany.

**Introduction.** Reactivation of latent viruses such as cytomegalovirus (CMV) may contribute to the initiation and progression of various autoimmune diseases. Efficient T cell immunity against CMV requires integrin-mediated adhesion of CMV-specific cytotoxic effector T cells to the endothelium or to virus-infected cells, which is induced by inside-out signaling following chemokine receptor or T cell receptor (TCR) stimulation, respectively. Previous analyses in healthy subjects indicated that epinephrine counteracts chemokine-induced inside-out signaling and in this way triggers de-adhesion of cytotoxic effector T cells from the endothelium.

**Methods.** To elucidate whether epinephrine suppresses integrin activity in TCR-stimulated cytotoxic T cells as well, we established a flow cytometric method that measures the binding of soluble multimeric intercellular adhesion molecule (ICAM)-1 complexes to beta2 integrins. CMV-specific T cells of healthy CMV-positive women and men were identified and stimulated using CMV peptide-major histocompatibility complex class I (pMHC) multimers in the presence or absence of epinephrine.

**Results** Within 2 minutes of TCR activation by CMV pMHC multimers ICAM-1 binding on CMV-specific cytotoxic T cells was significantly increased, indicating a rapid beta2 integrin activation. This process was counteracted by epinephrine in a dose-dependent manner. Interestingly, physiological levels of epinephrine were sufficient to suppress beta2 integrin activity. Unstimulated T cells showed no ICAM-1 binding.

**Conclusion.** Epinephrine suppresses integrin activity in CMV-stimulated cytotoxic T cells and presumably impairs target cell killing. This neuroendocrine influence on T cell immunity directed against CMV could explain CMV reactivation in stressful conditions and might play a role for CMV reactivation in autoimmune diseases.

# Loss of regulatory anti-Angiogenic Protease activated receptor-1 (PAR-1) Antibodies Associate with the Development of Metastatic Cancer Post Renal Transplantation and Patient Death

Dr. R. Catar[1,3], Dr. R. Carroll[2], I. Schramm[1], M. Simon[1], O. Wischnewski[1], Dr. A. Kusch[1], Dr. A. Philippe[1], Prof. Dr. D. Dragun[1,3]

[1]*Charite, Medizinische Klinik m.S. Nephrologie und Internistische Intensivmedizin - Berlin, Deutschland;* [2]*Royal Adelaide Hospital, Centre for Experimental Transplantation - Adelaide, Australien;* [3]*Berliner Institut für Gesundheitsforschung - Berlin, Deutschland*

**Introduction** Activated angiogenesis and impaired host immune response contribute to cancers in renal transplant recipients. Induction of VEGF is crucial for neoangiogenesis in tumors. Functional autoantibodies targeting GPCRs are able to induce endothelial dysfunction. We hypothesized that autoimmune GPCR targeting process may disturb VEGF induced angiogenesis. We identified in an in vitro model PAR-1 as a novel activating autoantibody target and assessed the presence of this naturally occurring blocking antibodies in 20 Kidney Transplant Recipients (KTR) with and 29 KTR without metastatic cancer.

**Methods** Human endothelial cells were stimulated with IgG isolated from sera of kidney transplant recipients (KTx-IgG). Transcriptional regulation of VEGF was studied by promoter deletion assay. Transcription factor activation and binding was assessed by qRT-PCR, western blot, EMSA and cFOS knockdown. VEGF secretion was determined by ELISA. Tube formation on matrigel served to study endothelial neoangiogenic response. All 49 patients enrolled had sera for assessment of PARab via ELISA in 2014 and at the time of transplantation.

**Results** Treatment with KTx-IgG reduced ERK1/2 dependent VEGF secretion and tube formation. VEGF secretion and endothelial tube formation could be only normalized by pretreatment with specific PAR-1 inhibitor. KTx-IgG contributed to deregulated neoangiogenesis via reduced VEGF-promoter activity and increased cFos protein expression via its binding to the VEGF promoter. PARab levels were lower at the time of transplant in KTR who developed cancer after transplant compared to those who did not. Levels were also different at the time of cancer diagnosis compared to those who had not developed cancer when assessed in 2014.

**Conclusions** We identified the PAR-1 receptor as a new target for functional antibodies in the context of kidney transplantation and tumor angiogenesis. PAR-1 regulated angiogenesis could offer new possibilities for treatment of kidney transplants obviate tumor angiogenesis.

# Imbalanced levels of circulating autoantibodies targeting muscarinic acetylcholine receptors in patients with systemic sclerosis

Sabine Sommerlatte[1], Silke Pitann[1], Mukaram Rana[1], Gabriele Marschner[1], Harald Heidecke[2], Jens Y Humrich[1], Tanja Lange[1], Peter Lamprecht[1], Antje Mueller[1], Otavio Cabral-Marques[1], Gabriela Riemekasten[1]

[1]Dept. of Rheumatology, University of Lübeck, Lübeck, Germany; [2]CellTrend GmbH, Luckenwalde, Brandenburg, Germany

**Introduction:** It has been shown that autoantibodies directed against G- protein coupled receptors (GPCRs) play a role in the pathogenesis of rheumatic diseases such as systemic sclerosis (SSc). Muscarinic acetylcholine receptors (mAChR) belong to the family of GPCRs and comprise five subtypes (M1-M5). They are part of the parasympathetic and central nervous system but are also expressed by immune cells and take part in the regulation of immune function. In addition, dysregulated levels of autoantibodies targeting mAChRs have been reported recently in patients with chronic fatigue syndrome (CFS). Fatigue is a frequent clinical manifestation in patients with SSc. However, whether those patients have imbalanced levels of autoantibodies targeting mAChRs compared to healthy controls (HCs) remains to be investigated.

**Methods:** Sera from patients with SSc (n = 42) and healthy controls (n = 42) were analyzed for the presence of autoantibodies recognizing muscarinic acetylcholine receptors (M1-5) using enzyme linked immunosorbent assay (ELISA).

**Results:** We found both elevated and reduced concentrations of circulating autoantibodies recognizing muscarinic acetylcholine receptors in SSc patients. In more detail, anti-M1 was elevated, while anti-M4 and -M5 were diminished compared to healthy controls. Concentrations of anti-M2 and –M3 did not significantly differ from those of healthy controls.

**Conclusion:** Imbalanced titers of autoantibodies targeting mAChRs may explain why fatigue is a frequent clinical manifestation in SSc patients. However, wheter the imbalanced levels of autoantibodies against mAChRs correlate with the occurrence and severity of fatigue in SSc patients needs to be further investigated.

# Dysregulated autoantibodies targeting complement receptors (C3aR, C5aR) & altered expression of C3aR and C5aR in rheumatic diseases

Sabine Sommerlatte[1], Silke Pitann[1], Mukaram Rana[1], Gabriele Marschner[1], Harald Heidecke[2], Jens Y Humrich[1], Tanja Lange[1], Peter Lamprecht[1], Antje Mueller[1], Otavio Cabral-Marques[1], Gabriela Riemekasten[1]

[1]Dept. of Rheumatology, University of Lübeck, Lübeck, Germany; [2]CellTrend GmbH, Luckenwalde, Brandenburg, Germany

**Introduction:** Autoantibodies targeting G-protein coupled receptors (GPCRS) are involved in the pathogenesis of rheumatic diseases such as systemic sclerosis (SSc). The superfamily of GPCRs comprises more than 1000 members, among them the complement receptors C3aR and C5aR. The complement system performs many functions, including regulation of inflammatory mechanisms. The aims of this study were to determine the concentrations of anti-C3aR and anti-C5aR in serum from patients with SSc, systemic lupus erythematosus (SLE), rheumatoid arthritis (RA), granulomatosis with polyangiitis (GPA) and healthy controls (HC) as well as the expression patterns of C3aR and C5aR by peripheral blood leukocyte (PBL) subpopulations, especially neutrophils (CD15+) and monocytes (CD14+) of the patients in comparison to HC. We hypothesize that autoantibodies targeting C3aR and C5aR are functionally active and regulate the corresponding ligand/receptor interactions.

**Methods:** Sera from patients with SLE (n☐45), SSc (n=73), RA (n☐76), GPA (n=38) and healthy controls (n≥175) were analyzed for the presence of autoantibodies targeting complement receptors C3aR and C5aR using enzyme linked immunosorbent assay (ELISA). After surface staining using anti-CD15, -CD14, -C3aR and -C5aR fluorochrome-conjugated antibodies the expression of C3aR and C5aR on PBLs subpopulations from patients (SLE=19, SSc=39, RA=21 and GPA=16) and healthy controls (HC=20) was analysed by flow cytometry.

**Results:** We found elevated anti-C3aR titers in SLE and reduced expression of C3aR on monocytes in SSc and on neutrophils in SSc, SLE, RA and GPA. Further, we observed a reduced concentration of anti-C5aR in SLE, SSc, RA and GPA. However, C5aR expression was not altered in any of the diseases.

**Conclusion:** The interplay between autoantibodies, receptors and the natural ligands C3a and C5a might be altered in rheumatic diseases. Thus, more studies are required to analyse if there are any correlations between anti-C3aR and/or anti-C5aR, ligand concentration and receptor expression, influencing functional effects of innate immune cells in rheumatic diseases.

# Loss of balance in circulating autoantibodies targeting CXCR3/CXCR4 and abnormal receptor expression on peripheral blood leukocytes in systemic lupus erythematosus

Mukaram Rana[1], Silke Pitann[1], Sabine Sommerlatte[1], Gabriele Marschner[1], Harald Heidecke[2], Jens Y Humrich[1], Peter Lamprecht[1], Antje Mueller[1], Otavio Cabral-Marques[1], Gabriela Riemekasten [1]

[1]Dept. of Rheumatology, University of Lübeck, Lübeck, Germany; [2]CellTrend GmbH, Luckenwalde, Brandenburg, Germany

**Background:** Aberrant cell migration and chemotaxis are pathophysiological mechanisms underlying vasculopathies in patients with systemic lupus erythematosus (SLE). However, the roles of the chemokine receptors CXCR3 and CXCR4 in SLE pathogenesis remain poorly explored.

**Aim:** To analyse the concentrations of circulating autoantibodies targeting CXCR3 and CXCR4, and the expression of these two receptors on peripheral blood leukocytes (PBL) from patients with SLE.

**Methods:** Anti-CXCR3 and anti-CXCR4 levels in sera from SLE patients (n = 249) were evaluated by ELISA in comparison to healthy controls (n = 198). Moreover, CXCR3 and CXCR4 expression on PBL from SLE patients (n = 10) and healthy subjects (n = 10) was evaluated by flow cytometry.

**Results:** Increased anti-CXCR3 and anti-CXCR4 autoantibodies concentrations were identified in SLE. Moreover, PBL subpopulations from SLE patients displayed alterations in CXCR3 and CXCR4 expression patterns. SLE patients demonstrated decreased CXCR3 expression on monocytes and CD4[+] T cells, while CXCR4 expression was increased on B and CD4[+] T cells.

**Conclusion:** SLE patients have increased circulating anti-CXCR3 and -CXCR4 antibody levels, which may be related to abnormal expression of CXCR3 and CXCR4 receptors. The mechanisms behind and consequent to these findings remain to be investigated.

# Effects of functional autoantibodies directed against angiotensin and endothelin receptors are influenced by the respective receptor expression

Judith Rademacher[1,2,3]*, Jeannine Günther[2,3], Elise Siegert[2,3], Angela Kill[2,3], Gabriela Riemekasten [4]

[1]Dept. of Rheumatology, Med. Department I, Campus Benjamin Franklin, Charité Universitätsmedizin Berlin, Germany; [2]Dept. of Rheumatology and Clinical Immunology, Charité University Hospital, Berlin, Germany; [3]Cell Autoimmunity Group, German Rheumatism Research Center (DRFZ), Berlin, Germany; [4]Dept. of Rheumatology, University of Lübeck, Lübeck, Germany;

**Introduction**: Functional autoantibodies against angiotensin II receptor type 1 (AT1R) and endothelin-1 receptor type A (ETAR) are elevated in patients with systemic sclerosis (SSc) and induce the production of cytokines such as the profibrotic CCL18 and interleukin 8 (IL-8). We analyzed whether protein expression of the respective receptors as well as their functional counterparts AT2R and ETBR influences the effects of these autoantibodies in SSc patients and healthy donors.

**Methods**: AT1R, AT2R, ETAR and ETBR protein expression on peripheral blood mononuclear cells (PBMC) of SSc patients and healthy donors was measured by flow cytometry and correlated with clinical data. PBMC of healthy donors were *in vitro* stimulated with immunglobulin G (IgG) of patients and healthy donors. IL-8 and CCL18 cytokine concentration was then quantified in the supernatants by enzyme-linked immunosorbent assay and correlated with receptor expression of the stimulated PBMC.

**Results**: Angiotensin and Endothelin Receptor expression on PBMC of patients with SSc was elevated compared to age-and sex-matched healthy donors, while AT1R/AT2R ratio was increased. ETAR/ETBR correlated with clinical manifestations of the disease such as lung and skin fibrosis. CCL18 and IL-8 cytokine induction by SSc-IgG and HD-IgG was influenced by the receptor expression and respective ratios. IL-8 secretion correlated negatively with the AT1R/AT2R ratio and positively with the ETAR/ETBR ratio of the stimulated PBMC.

**Conclusion**: Angiotensin and endothelin receptor expression and the ratio of the receptor subtypes influence autoantibody-mediated effects such as the production of the profibrotic cytokines IL-8 and CCL-18. Receptor expression might thereby play a crucial role in autoimmunity.

## Antibodies to signaling molecules and receptors relate to apoptosis and inflammation in heart failure

Anders Lund, *Medical Student**[1], Lasse M. Giil, *MD*[1,2], Einar Kristoffersen, *MD, PhD*[1,3], Christian Vedeler, *MD, PhD*[4], Ralf Dechend, *MD, PhD*[5,6], Gabriela Riemekasten, MD, PhD[7] Harald Heidecke, *MScPharm, PhD*[8], Jan Erik Nordrehaug, *MD, PhD*[1]

[1]*Department of Clinical Science, University of Bergen, Bergen, Norway;* [2]*Department of Internal Medicine, Haraldsplass Deaconess Hospital, Bergen, Norway;* [3]*Department of Immunology and Transfusion Medicine, Haukeland University Hospital, Bergen, Norway;* [4]*Institute of Clinical Medicine, University of Bergen, Bergen, Norway;* [5]*HELIOS-Klinikum Berlin-Buch, Berlin, Germay;* [6]*Experimental and Clinical Research Center, Charité Medical Faculty and the Max-Delbruck Center for Molecular Medicine, Berlin, Germany;* [7]*Department of Rheumatology, University Hospital Schleswig-Holstein, Lübeck, Germany;* [8]*CellTrend GmbH, Luckenwalde, Berlin, Germany*

**Background.** Antibodies to signaling molecules and receptors form networks of correlated antibodies to multiple receptors, even in healthy individuals. Physiological antibodies have been linked to inflammation and apoptosis, both important pathophysiological processes in heart failure (HF). We investigated if there is a link between antibodies to a broad range of signaling molecules and receptors and biomarkers of inflammation and apoptosis.

**Methods.** Antibodies (ab) in pre-analytically randomized sera from patients ($n=202$) with ischemic cardiomyopathy (ICM) ($n = 166$) and non-ICM ($n = 36$) were measured with full-receptor sandwich enzyme-linked immunosorbent assays. Non-parametric statistics were used for analysis of association, reported as effect size ($r$) and corrected for multiple testing. Troponin-T (TNT) elevation not due to ischemia was used as a marker for myocardial apoptosis. C reactive protein (CRP), leukocyte count, kynurenine-tryptophan ratio, (KTR, a marker of interferon-$\gamma$ activity), fibrinogen (coagulation and inflammation) and neopterin (a marker of activated monocytes) were measured as immune-markers.

**Results.** TNT correlated with Stabilin1-ab ($r$ 0.29, p < 0.001). CRP correlated with soluble endoglin-ab (sENG-ab, $r$ 0.20, p = 0.01), fibrinogen with sENG-ab ($r$ 0.28, p < 0.001), neopterin with platelet-derived growth factor β-ab ($r$ 0.27, p < 0.001). There were both positive (dopamin D2s receptor, $r$ 0.26, p < 0.001) and negative (soluble pro-renin receptor, $r$ -0.32, p < 0,001) correlations with KTR.

**Conclusion.** Antibodies to vascular and immune-related receptors were correlated with apoptosis and innate immune activation in patients with predominantly ICM. These processes, linked to physiological antibodies, are also important mediators of disease progression in HF. Both endoglin and the pro-renin receptors are linked to myocardial fibrosis. Depending on which effects these antibodies have on their receptor-antigens, they could provide new links to key pathophysiological processes in HF.

www.ingramcontent.com/pod-product-compliance
Lightning Source LLC
Chambersburg PA
CBHW081554220326
41598CB00036B/6667